QUICK-E

Med-Surg

Second Edition

Medical Surgical
Clinical Nursing Reference

Martin Schiavenato RN, BSN, MS

BANDIDO BOOKS

Copyright © 2002 by Bandido Books All rights reserved
Printed in the United States of America

Copyright © 2002 by Bandido Books. All rights reserved
Although the author and publisher have exhaustively researched numerous sources to ensure the accuracy and completeness of the information contained in this book, we assume no responsibility for errors, inaccuracies, ommissions or any other inconsistency herein.

"Martin's Quick-E" is a trademark ™ of Bandido Books. No part of this book may be reproduced by any electronic or mechanical means without written permission from the publisher

Includes references. Orlando, Florida 2002

ISBN 1-929693-17-6

Other fine titles available in the *Quick-E* Series:

- **I.V.** *Intravenous Nursing*
- **E.R.** *Emergency Nursing*
- **Peds** *Pediatric Nursing*
- **O.B** *Obstetric Nursing*
- **Med-Surg** *Medical Surgical*
- **Assessment** *& Physical Exam*
- **Charting** *& Terminology*
- **Spanish Guide for Nurses**
- **Dysrhythmia Recognition**
- **Critical Care**

To keep abreast of changes, additions and new products, please visit us at **www.bandidobooks.com** or contact us via email at *publish@bandidobooks.com* or by postal service at:

Bandido Books | 9806 Heaton Court | Orlando, FL 32817

Happy Nursing!

Nursing at Clinical Speed!

To order call our Toll-Free Hotline at 1-877-814-6824 PIN 1174

Reviewers

Angeline Bushy PhD, RN, CS
Professor, Bert Fish Endowed Chair
University of Central Florida, School of Nursing
Daytona Campus, Florida

Robert S. Jacobs RN, BSN
Staff Nurse, Emergency Department
Satilla Regional Medical Center
Waycross, Georgia

Denise Tucker RN, DSN, CCRN
Associate in Nursing
Florida State University, School of Nursing
Tallahassee, Florida

Kevin M. Wilks RNC, MSN
Nursing Instructor Supervisor
Eleanor Slater Hospital
Cranston, Rhode Island

*To Tulls and Squito,
my life.*

M.S.

This reference work is designed to be used by qualified licensed professionals and, or students under the supervision of a qualified professional. The publisher assumes no responsibilities or liabilities from any effects of the implementation of the information imparted here, nor from any undetected errors or reader misunderstanding of the text. For their protection, readers are urged to practice within their scope as prescribed by the regional professional governing body and, or the local institution. This work is not intended to supersede or replace any rules, policies or standards of practice applicable to the user.

Contents

Section Color Code Scheme. **Green:** Lab Values, Units of Measurement, Hormone Guide, Infection Control, Assessment **Blue:** IV Therapy, Nutrition **Red:** BLS, Medications **Gray:** Nursing Diagnoses and Reference

Lab Values
1 CBC, Chemistry
2 Sedimentation Rate, Coagulation Studies, Cardiac profile
3 Urine, Fecal Studies, Drug Levels, ABGs and Using Lab Values

Units of Measurement
4 Temperature and Weight Conversion Tables, Equivalents of Measurements

Hormone Guide
5-8 Organ, Hormone and Effect

Infection Control
9 Universal Precautions
10 Bloodborne Pathogens: Occupational Exposure

Assessment
11 Abdominopelvic Quadrants, Assessment Scales
12 Cranial Nerves
13 Neurologic Reference
14 Breath Sounds, Chest Tubes
15 Oxygen Delivery Systems, Cardiac Assessment, Heart Sounds, Murmur Scales
16 Auscultatory Areas, Pacemaker Terminology, Pacemaker Codes
17 Bowel Sounds, Pressure Sore Scale
18 *Quick-E* 5 minute assessment

Intravenous Therapy
19 Site Assessment, Infiltration Scale, Phlebitis Scale
20 Catheter Gauge Selection, Tonicity and Fluids

Nutrition
21 Feeding Tubes
22 Feeding Tube Complications and Management
23 Recommended Daily Dietary Allowances (RDAs)
24 Determining Body Mass Index (BMI)
25 Estimating Ideal Body Weight (IBW), Relative Health Risk by BMI and Waist Size
26, 27 Vitamins: Source and Action

Basic Life Support (BLS)
29, 30 Cardiopulmonary Resuscitation (CPR)
31, 32 Automated External Defibrillator (AED)

Medications
33 Dosage Formulas
34 Syringe Compatibility
35 Commonly Used Analgesics in Adults, Insulin Preparations

Nursing Diagnoses
37-39 NANDA Nursing Diagnoses
40 References

Author's Preface

This book, as others in the *Quick-E Series*, is intended to be used by nurses and nursing students as a quick, portable, and easy-to-use pocket reference. The goal of this volume is not to be exhaustive in its clinical content to the areas of medical-surgical nursing, but rather to provide clinicians with easy access to often-needed information in a clinical setting.

Quick-E: Med-Surg aims to maximize the nurse's time by facilitating information in a durable and portable format ideal for the "bedside" practice. Ultimately, my intent is that this book helps to enhance the quality of patient care through quick access to clinical facts applicable and usable in the medical-surgical practice.

The book is organized by topical content separated by color dividers to facilitate quick location of information. The color dividers are placed throughout the text to help the user thumb through pages and to quickly identify sections and locate material. For the sake of brevity and practicality certain abbreviations and symbols are used throughout the text and assume a basic knowledge of medical terminology by the user. Users are strongly encouraged to adhere to institutional standards in obtaining, interpreting, applying and documenting all clinical findings. Since all individual clinical practice is unique, I have added room throughout the text for you to customize this tool with your own clinical notes. Additional information and more in-depth clinical and academic coverage may be found in the "Reference" section.

Happy Nursing!

Laboratory Values*

CBC

RBC	4.7-6.1 million/mm³ (♂) 4.2-5.4 million/mm³ (♀)	Hgb	13.5-17.5 g/dl (♂) 12-16 g/dl (♀)
WBC	4300-10800 cells/mm³	Hct	40-54 % (♂) 37-47 % (♀)
Platelets	150-350 thousand/mm³	MCV	80-94 cu microns
MCH	27-32 pg	MCHC	32-36 %

Chemistry

Na	135-148 mEq/L	K	3.5-5.0 mEq/L
Cl	98-106 mEq/L	CO_2	24-32 mEq/L
BUN	7-18 mg/dl	Uric Acid	3.0-7.0 mg/dl
Ca	8.5-10.5 mg/dl	Mg	1.3-2.1 mEq/L
Creatinine	0.7-1.3 mg/dl (♂) 0.6-1.2 mg/dl (♀)	Glucose (fasting)	70-110 mg/dl
Bilirubin Direct 0-0.2 mg/dl Total 0.2-1.0 mg/dl Indirect Total minus Direct		SGPT (ALT)	10-55 U/L (♂) 7-30 U/L (♀)
Osmolality	275-295 mOsm/kg	Anion gap	8-16 mEg/L
Amylase	50-150 U/L	Lipase	4-24 U/L
Alkaline Phosphatase (ALP) 13-39 U/L (adults)		Lipids	See page 27 "Cholesterol Recommendations"

*Refers to adult values unless otherwise noted

"It's better to be sick than nurse the sick. Sickness is single trouble for the sufferer; but nursing means vexation of the mind, and hard work for the hands besides."

Euripedes

Sedimentation Rate

Wintrobe 0-9 mm per hour (♂) 0-20 mm per hour (♀)	*Westergren* 1-13 mm per hour (♂) 1-20 mm per hour (♀)

Coagulation

PT	10-14 sec	**PTT**	30-45 sec
APTT	16-25 sec	**ACT**	92-128 sec
FSP	<10 μg/dl	**Platelets**	150-350 thousand/mm^3

Cardiac Profile

SGOT (AST)	7-21 U/L (♂) 6-18 U/L (♀)	**SGOT** *with MI*	Onset 12-18 hours Peak 24-48 hours Duration 3-4 days
CK	38-174 U/L (♂) 96-140 U/L (♀)	**CK** *with MI*	Onset 4-6 hours Peak 12-24 hours Duration 3-4 days
CK-MB	0 %	**CK-MB** *with MI*	Onset 4-6 hours Peak 12-24 hours Duration 2-3 days
LDH	90-200 U/L	**LDH** *with MI*	Onset 24-48 hours Peak 3-6 days Duration 7-10 days
LDH$_1$ **LDH$_2$**	17.5-28.3% total LDH 30.4-36.4% total LDH	*With MI*	LDH$_1$ > LDH$_2$ Onset 12-24 hours Peak 48 hours Duration Variable
Troponin I At least 1.5μg/ml to 3.1μg/ml for AMI (acute myocardial Infarction)		**Myoglobin** References varying for AMI from 50 μg/ml to 120μg/ml	

Urine Values

Specific Gravity	1.003-1.030	PH	4.5-8.0
Osmolality	300-1200 mOsm/L	Volume	1200 (600-2500cc/24hrs)
Glucose	Normally not found	Protein	Normally not found
Bilirubin	Negative	Urobilinogen	Up to 1.0 Ehrlich U

❖ *Consistent appearance of* casts *and* epithelial cells *is abnormal*

Fecal Studies

Occult Blood (FOBT, hemoccult, guaiac)	Negative
Trypsin Positive result is normal	Ova and Parasites Negative

Drug Levels

Digoxin 1-2 ng/ml	Phenytoin 10-20 mcg/ml
Theophylline 10-20 mcg/ml	Barbiturate coma 10 mg/100ml
Gentamicin Trough 1-2 mcg/ml Peak 6-8 mcg/ml	Tobramycin Trough 1-2 mcg/ml Peak 6-8 mcg/ml

ABG'S

PH	7.35-7.45	Pao$_2$	80-100 mm Hg
Paco$_2$	35-45 mm Hg	HCO$_3$	22-26 mEq/L
% Sat	95-99	Base Excess	+/-2

Using Lab Values

To assess status:	Consult:
Renal	Urine values, BUN, creatinine, serum electrolytes
Liver	ALP, SGPT, bilirubin (serum and urine), urobilinogen, LDH, PT, cholesterol, hepatitis profile
Pancreatic	Amylase, lipase
Respiratory	ABG'S, sputum culture
Cardiac	See *Cardiac Profile*, lipids

"A little rebellion now and then is a good thing."
Thomas Jefferson

Units of Measurement

Temperature

$°F - 32 \times 0.5555 = °C$		$°C \times 1.8 + 32 = °F$	
°F	°C	°C	°F
0	-17.8	0	32.0
95	35.0	35.0	95.0
96	35.6	35.5	95.9
97	36.1	36.0	96.8
98	36.7	36.5	97.7
99	37.2	37.0	98.6
100	37.8	37.5	99.5
101	38.3	38.0	100.4
102	38.9	38.5	101.3
103	39.4	39.0	102.2
104	40.0	39.5	103.1
105	40.6	40.0	104.0

Weight

$lbs / 2.2 = Kgs$		$Kgs \times 2.2 = lbs$	
lb	Kg	Kg	lb
1	0.5	1	2.2
2	0.9	2	4.4
4	1.8	5	11
10	4.5	10	22
50	22.7	50	110
100	45.5	80	176
150	68.2	90	198
200	90.9	100	220

Equivalents of Measurement

Metric (volume)	Apothecary	Household
1 ml	15 minims	15 drops
15 ml	4 fluidrams	1 tablespoon
30 ml	1 fluid ounce	2 tablespoons
240 ml	8 fluid ounces	1 cup
480 ml (approx. ½ L)	1 pint	1 pint
960 ml (approx. 1 L)	1 quart	1 quart
3840 ml	1 gallon	1 gallon

Hormone Guide

Organ	Hormone	Effect
Adrenal {adrenal cortex} {adrenal medulla}	Mineralocorticoids (mainly aldosterone but over 2 dozen produced)	↑Na and ↓K; ↑water and BP. *Hyposecretion: Addison's. Hypersecretion: Aldosteronism*
	Glucocorticoids (mainly cortisol)	Blood sugar levels, fat metabolism, protein catabolism, assists body to resist stressors, depress inflamatory and immune responses. *Hyposecretion: Addison's. Hypersecretion: Cushing's*
	Gonadocorticoids (sex hormones, mainly androgens)	Thought to affect ♀ sex drive and provide small amounts of estrogen after menopause
	Epinephrine and noroepinephrine	AKA catecholamines. Sympathetic nervous system. Flight-or-fight. Epi ↑heart and metabolic activities and bronchodilation, noroepi ↑peripheral vasoconstriction.
Gonads (♂ testes, ♀ ovaries)	♀ Estrogen and progesterone	Secondary sex characteristics, maturation of reproductive organs, estrogen promotes uterine changes in menstrual cycle
	♂ Testosterone	Secondary sex characteristics, maturation of reproductive organs, sperm production

Organ	Hormone	Effect
Pancreas	Glucagon	Hyperglycemic agent. *Persisten low blood sugar levels may be associated with glucagon deficiency*
	Insulin	Lowers blood sugar level and influences protein and fat metabolism. *Hyposecretion: Diabete mellitus. Hyperinsulinism may occur and is commonly from an overdose of insulin*
Parathyroid	Parathyroid hormone	Ca balance. *Surgical removal of gland may result in hypocalcemia, tetany, sizure and death if not corrected*
Pineal	Melatonin	Inhibits gonadotropic functions, sleep/wake cycle
Pituitary	Growth hormone	Body growth, protein and fat metabolism. *Hyposecretion: Pituitary dwarfism. Hypersecretion: giantism (children), acromegaly (adults).*
	Thyroid stimulating hormone (TSH)	Growth and maintenance of thyroid gland
	Adrenocorticotropic hormone (ACTH)	Growth and maintenance of adrenal cortex
	Prolactin	Milk secretion, maintenance of corpus luteum
	Follicle stimulating hormone (FSH) and luteinizing hormone (LH), referred to as gonadotropins	Regulate function of gonads (both ♂ and ♀)

Organ	Hormone	Effect
Pituitary (cont.)	Oxytocin	Uterine contraction and ejection of milk
	Antidiuretic hormone (ADH)	Inhibits urine formation. *Hyposecretion: Diabetes insipidus, most commonly from hypothalmic trauma*
Thymus	Thymopoietin, thymosin	Primary central gland of the lymphatic system. T cells develop here, essential for development of normal immune response
Thyroid *(goiter: enlarged thyroid gland)*	Thyroxine T_4, triiodothyronine T_3	↑Rate of cellular metabolism in body (BMR). Affects virtually every cell in the body, regulates tissue growth and development, nervous system development and reproductive capabilities. Plays a role in BP maintenance, and temperature regulation. *Hyposecretion: Myxedema (in children, severe hypothyrodism: Cretinism). Hypersecretion: Grave's.*
	Calcitonin	Antagonist of parathyroid hormone, ↓blood Ca levels

"I have always held firmly to the thought that each one of us can do a little to bring some portion of misery to an end."
Albert Schweitzer

Organ	Hormone	Effect
Other	Prostaglandins (associated with plasma membrane)	Mediate hormone responses, stimulates smooth muscles of arterioles or uterus, ↑HCl and pepsin secretion by stomach, ↑inflamation and pain, induce fever
	Gastrin (stomach), enterogastrin, secretin, cholecystokinin (duodenum)	Regulate secretion of HCl, bicarbonate, and digestive enzymes
	Erythropoietin (kidney)	Act on bone marrow to ↑RBC production
	Atrial natriuretic factor (atrium of heart)	↓BP

"There never was a good war or a bad peace."
Benjamin Franklin

Notes:

Infection Control
Universal (Standard) Precautions

- The CDC defines universal (standard) precautions as "a set of precautions designed to prevent transmission of human immunodeficiency virus (HIV), hepatitis B virus (HBV), hepatitis C virus (HBV), and other bloodborne pathogens"*

- All patients are potential sources of infectious diseases

- Gloves are considered the minimal barrier. Gloves will not protect you from injury from sharp objects. Gloves should always be changed after contact with patient, and hands should be washed immediately after removal of gloves

- If the generation of droplets, or splashing of blood or body fluids is anticipated during therapy/procedure, additional protective barriers should be worn (gowns, masks, goggles)

- Dispose of blood-contaminated items properly, and again, assume that they are potentially infectious

- Utilize needleless, or safety-engineered products in accordance with manufacturer's instructions and facility policy

- Dispose of sharps properly and carefully (do not over-stuff containers to prevent breakage of materials and injury; follow manufacturer's instructions for filling limits, and correct handling)

- Follow product instructions to maintain product sterility. Maintain aseptic technique with infusion procedures. Remember: *hand washing is the primary infection control measure*

* *Hospital Infectious Program*. National Center for Infectious Diseases, Center for Disease Control and Prevention. 1999

Bloodborne Pathogens: Occupational Exposure

• **Hepatitis B (HBV)** Transmitted by percutaneous or mucosal exposure to blood and serum derived body fluids from infected individuals. Vaccine is available and recommended. Vaccine should be offered to exposed, unvaccinated person and, if exposure source is known to be positive, hepatitis B immune globulin (HBIG) should be given as treatment (tx), preferably within 24 hrs of exposure. Risk of infection for unvaccinated person: 6-30%

• **Hepatitis C (HCV)** Most common chronic bloodborne infection in the US. Most individuals are chronically infected and do not know about it since they show no clinical signs or symptoms. Virus is transmitted primarily through large or repeated direct percutaneous exposures to blood. Immune globulin and antiviral agents (e.g., interferon with or without ribavirin) are not recommended for post-exposure prophylaxes of hepatitis C. No vaccine is available. Risk of infection approximately 1.8% for needle stick or cut (risk from a blood splash unknown but believed to be small)

• **Human Immunodeficiency Virus (HIV)** As of printing, no vaccine is available although many are currently being researched. Prophylactic tx is not recommended for all occupational exposures to HIV because most exposures do not lead to infection, and the tx drugs may have serious side effects. Decision for tx should be taken in consultation of health care provider. Current tx recommendations include a basic 4-week regimen of two drugs (zidovudine [ZDV] and lamivudine [3TC]; 3TC and stavudine [d4T]; or didanosine [ddI] and d4T) for most HIV exposures and an expanded regimen that includes the addition of a third drug for HIV exposures that pose an increased risk for transmission. Recommendations are guidelines and may be modified clinically as needed. Risk of infection from needle stick or cut is 0.3%. Risk after exposure of the eye, nose or mouth to HIV infected blood is 0.1%. Risk after exposure of the skin to HIV infected blood is < 0.1%

Assessment

Abdominopelvic Quadrants

Right Upper Quadrant
Liver
Gallbladder
Pylorus
Head of pancreas
Duodenum
Upper right kidney

Right Lower Quadrant
Lower right kidney
Cecum
Appendix
Ascending colon
R fallopian tube (♀)
R ovary (♀)
R ureter, Bladder (distended)

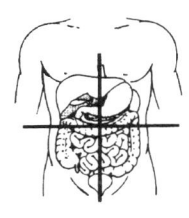

Left Upper Quadrant
Left lobe of liver
Spleen
Stomach
Body of pancreas
Left kidney

Left Lower Quadrant
Descending colon
Sigmoid colon
L ureter
Bladder (distended)
L fallopian tube (♀)
L ovary (♀)

Assessment Scales

Pitting Edema		Pulse	
+1	5mm depth	0	Absent
+2	8-10 mm depth	+1	Decreased, thready
+3	> 10 mm depth, up to 30 sec	+2	Normal
+4	>20 mm depth, longer than 30 sec	+3	Full, bounding
Deep Tendon Reflexes		**Muscle Movement of Extremities**	
0	Absent	0	No contraction
1+	Diminished	1	Slight contraction
2+	Normal	2	Active with gravity eliminated
3+	Increased	3	Active with gravity
4+	Hyperactive, clonus	4	Active, some resistance
		5	Full strength against resistance

Cranial Nerves

Cranial Nerve	Type	Function	Assessment
I Olfactory	Sensory	Smell	Test with non-noxious smells such as orange, coffee, soap or vanilla
II Optic	Sensory	Vision	Visual acuity
III Oculomotor	Mixed	Ocular movement, pupil constriction, lens shape, eyelids	Check pupils for size, light reaction and accommodation.
IV Trochlear	Motor	Eye movement	Assess extraocular movements
V Trigeminal	Mixed	Chewing, sensation of face, cornea, scalp, mouth and nose	Palpate chewing muscles as client clenches teeth. Check for sensation on face
VI Abducens	Motor	Lateral eye movement	*
VII Facial	Mixed	Taste on anterior tongue, facial muscles, close eye, saliva, tears	Lift eyebrows, smile. Identify taste of safe substance (lemon, salt)
VIII Acoustic	Sensory	Hearing and balance	Hearing acuity
IX Glossopharyngeal	Mixed	Gag reflex, taste on posterior tongue, swallowing, parotid gland, carotid reflex	Assess uvula and soft palate placement with tongue depress while client says "ahh."
X Vagus	Mixed	Talking and swallowing, general carotid sensation, sinus, and reflex	Uvula to midline. Note gag reflex.
XI Spinal	Motor	Trapezius and sternomastoid movement	Shrug shoulders. Rotate head to sides against resistance.
XII Hypoglossal	Motor	Tongue movement	Note speech. Midline forward thrust of tongue

* Assessed together with cranial nerves III and IV

Neurologic Reference

Sign	Description
Babinski	Sole of foot is stroked. Abnormal: Dorsiflexion of big toe and fanning of the toes Upper motor neuron dysfunction. Normal: Plantar flexion
Brudzinski	Passive neck flexion trigger flexion of the hip and knee. Pathologic reflex indicating meningeal irritation
Kernig	Resistance to full extension of the leg at the knee when the hip is flexed. Pathologic reflex indicating meningeal irritation
Oculocephalic (doll's eye maneuver)	Head rotated from side to side. Abnormal: Eyes move with the head fixed in place. This is a normal response in newborns but disappears as ocular fixation develops. Indicates brainstem injury. Normal: Eyes remain in the initial position, then turn slowly in the direction of head rotation
Oculovestibular (ice water calorics, also called Barany's test)	Ear alternately irrigated with hot and cold water. Abnormal: *Supratentorial or metabolic lesion*, eyes move slowly toward irrigated ear and remain there for 2-3 minutes. Absent fast return to midline. *Brainstem lesion*, downward deviation and rotary jerking of one eye. *Severe brainstem injury*, no response. Normal: Hot water irrigation produces a rotatory nystagmus towards irrigated ear. Cold water produces a rotatory nystagmus away from irrigated ear
Decorticate	Flexion of upper extremities, legs may be extended. Indicates lesion to the mesencephalic region of the brain
Decerebrate	Extension of upper extremities with internal rotation, legs may be extended. Indicates brainstem lesion

- **Spinal Cord** 31 Pairs of spinal nerves originate from the cord: 8 cervical, 12 thoracic, 5 lumbar, 5 sacral, 1 coccygeal. Lesions below first thoracic vertebra may produce *paraplegia*. Lesions above first thoracic vertebra may produce *quadriplegia*. Lesions that completely transect the spinal cord cause loss of motor and sensory function below the level of injury.

- **Dysreflexia** state in which an individual with a spinal cord injury at T7 or above experiences a life threatening uninhibited sympathetic response of the nervous system to a noxious stimulus. S+S include pallor below the injury, red splotches on skin above the injury, paroxysmal hypertension (sudden periodic ↑BP systolic >140 and diastolic >90mm Hg), headache, blurred vision, chest pain, horner's syndrome, metallic taste in mouth, gooseflesh formation when skin is cooled. Treatment: Elevate head, identify and remove noxious stimulus (bladder or bowel distention, skin irritation etc), monitor BP closely, have available antihypertensives as physician prescribes

Breath Sounds

❖ Auscultate in a systematic manner both anterior and posterior chest walls starting from the apices and working from side to side, downward to bases. Do not auscultate over bone or breast tissue.

Adventitious Sounds

Crackles	Air that contains serous secretions. Bubbling, wet sound (a.k.a. rales). Pneumonia, CHF, bronchitis, emphysema
Wheezes	Air flowing through narrow airways. High pitch, musical quality. Acute asthma, bronchitis
Stridor	High pitch, crowing sound. Croup, airway obstruction, acute epiglotitis (children)
Rub	Coarse and low pitch. Pleuritis

Assess

Pitch	Is it high or low?
Timing	When is it occurring? Late or early? Inspiratory or expiratory?
Quality	Is it loud or soft? Coarse or fine? Is it continuous or intermittent?
Location	Where on the chest wall was sound auscultated?

Chest Tube Drainage

Water Seal Chamber	Collection Chamber	Suction Chamber
Usual level at 2-3 cm. Bubbling indicates air leak in system. If bubbling, clamp near client. If bubbling stops, leak within client or at insertion site. Notify physician. If bubbling does not stop, leak is in the system. Locate leak by clamping along tubing. Replace and retape equipment prn	If drainage >100 ml/hr for 2 hours or sudden change in amount of bloody drainage, notify physician. If drainage is decreased, check for kinks and clots. Consult your local protocol in regards to milking tube	Usual 15-25 cm water. Maintain constant, gentle bubbling. Maintain appropriate fluid level. ❦ Keep a bottle of sterile water and sterile petroleum gauze available. If system interrupted, tube should be placed in a few cms of sterile water while system reestablished. Gauze for applying to chest wall if tube is accidentally removed

Oxygen Delivery Systems

Nasal Cannula	4-6 L/min deliver 35-40% FIO_2. Higher flow rates dry airway mucosa and not recommended
Simple Mask	Minimum flow of 5-6 L/min. 10-12 L/min deliver 55-65% FIO_2
Nonrebreathing Mask	Attached reservoir allows theoretical delivery of 90-100% FIO_2. In practice, usually delivers up to 70% FIO_2 at 10 L/min
Venturi Mask	Delivers controlled FIO_2 at specific rates. 4 L/min (24%), 6 L/min (28%), 8 L/min (35%) and 10 L/min (40% FIO_2)

Cardiac Assessment

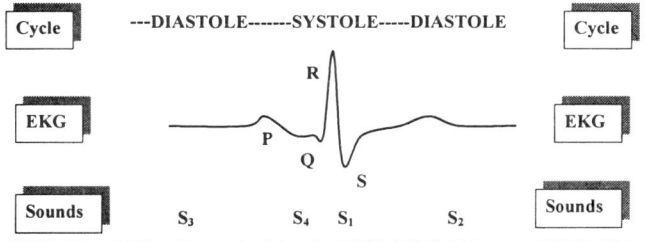

---DIASTOLE-------SYSTOLE-----DIASTOLE

EKG: P, Q, R, S

Sounds: S_3 S_4 S_1 S_2

Murmur Scale

Grade	Description
I	Barely audible
II	Audible
III	Moderately loud, no thrill
IV	Loud, no thrill
V	Very loud, associated with a thrill
VI	Very loud, thrill, audible with Stethoscope off the chest

Heart Sounds

S_1	Beginning systole. Loudest at apex. Caused by closure of AV valves
S_2	Loudest at base. Caused by closure of semilunar valves
S_3	May be normal when in children and young adults. Associated with CHF. Abnormal over age 35 termed *ventricular gallop*
S_4	May occur in adults >40 without disease. Pathologic S_4 termed *atrial gallop*

Auscultatory Areas

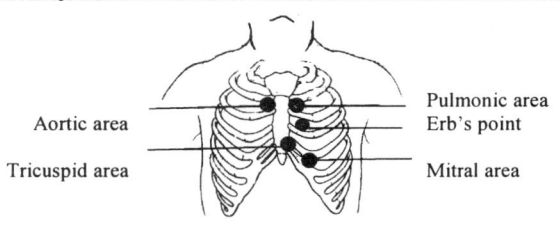

Aortic area

Tricuspid area

Pulmonic area

Erb's point

Mitral area

❖ Erbs's point is frequently the area to which aortic or pulmonic sounds radiate. Valve areas are not over actual anatomic sites but are where sounds produced by the valves are best heard

Pacemaker Terminology

Fixed-rate *(asynchronous)* Paces at fixed rate regardless of spontaneous cardiac activity

Demand *(synchronous)* Paces only when heart's intrinsic pacemaker fails to function at a predetermined rate.

AV Sequential *(dual-chamber pacing)* Paces both atrium and ventricle in sequence

Pacemaker Codes

Code	Description	Code	Description
AOO	Atrial (A) fixed rate, no sensing	AAT	A demand, paced/sensed, triggered response to sensing
VOO	Ventricular (V) fixed rate, no sensing	VAT	AV synchronous, V pacing, A sensing, triggered response
DOO	AV sequential fixed, no sensing	DVI	AV sequential, A+V pacing, V sensing, inhibited response
VVI	V demand, V paced/sensed, inhibited response to sensing	VDD	A synchronous, V inhibited, V pacing, A+V sensing, inhibited response to sensing in V and triggered response to sensing in A
VVT	V demand, V paced/sensed, triggered response to sensing		
AAI	A demand, paced/sensed, inhibited response to sensing	DDD	Universal, A+V senses and paced inhibited in V, triggered in A

Bowel Sounds

Normal	5-3 times per minute
Hyperactive	Loud, high pitch, rushing, tinkling sounds. Borborygmus (stomach growling), signal increased motility. Occur with early mechanical bowel obstruction (high pitched), gastroenteritis, brisk diarrhea, laxative use, subsiding paralytic ileus
Hypoactive	Signal decreased motility due to inflammation. Occur with peritonitis, paralytic ileus as following abdominal surgery, and late bowel obstruction. Also occurs with pneumonia and electrolyte imbalance. A "silent" abdomen is uncommon. Listen for 5 minutes before deciding that bowel sounds are completely absent

Pressure Sore Scale*

Stage I	Non-blanchable erythema of intact skin; indicates likely progression to ulceration
Stage II	Partial thickness skin loss; involves epidermis and/or dermis. This superficial ulcer appears as an abrasion, blister, or shallow crater
Stage III	Full-thickness skin loss; involves subcutaneous tissue and may extend down to (but excludes) the fascia. This deeper ulcer appears as a deep crater and may have undermining of adjacent tissues
Stage IV	Full-thickness skin loss with destruction of tissue including the muscle, bone, or supporting structures. Undermining of adjacent structures may be present

* Wounds covered with eschar may not be staged unless the eschar is removed to determine the extent of underlying tissue destruction/necrosis. Never "de-stage" a pressure sore as it heals, i.e. a Stage III sore later becomes a "healing Stage III sore" *not* a Stage II or Stage I sore

Quick E Head-To-Toe 5 Minute Assessment

- Gather and review hx and meds from chart, kardex or report
- General appearance (loc, gait, mood, affect, speech, hearing, *how are you feeling, what is bothering you?*)
- Head and neck (eye contact, pupils, skin condition, scalp, lips and tongue, cervical lymph nodes, neck vessels, *trouble swallowing, poor appetite, drinking O.K.?*)
- Upper extremities (patent pulses bilaterally, skin temp and turgor, grasp, ROM, *any pain or trouble moving?*)
- Anterior and posterior chest wall (inspect, palpate and auscultate). Listen for extra heart sounds, murmurs Note heart rate and rhythm. Listen for adventitious breath sounds, *any chest pain or difficulty breathing?*
- Abdomen (first inspect, then auscultate, then palpate) Note bowel sounds, presence of abdominal rigidity or enlarged organs. Light palpation first followed by deeper palpation, *any pain, are bowels moving fine, are you voiding O.K.?*
- Lower extremities (patent pulses bilaterally, skin temp and turgor, capillary refill, assess strength by asking to push ball of foot against your hand, ROM, note any edema, *any problems moving, any calf tenderness?*

Italics are questions for client. Refer to other portions of the book for specific techniques.

> *"Any sufficiently advanced technology is indistinguishable from magic."*
> Arthur C. Clarke

Intravenous Therapy

Site Assessment

Color	Redness, blanching, translucence, discoloration?
Look for	Hematoma, bruising, swelling, streak formation, leakage, bleeding, purulent drainage, tissue necrosis
Feel for	Cording, skin tightness, pitting, induration. Assess for presence of pain, numbness and circulatory impairment (capillary refill, pulse)

Infiltration Scale

Value	Interpretation
0	No clinical symptoms
1	Skin blanched. *Edema < 1 inch.* Cool to touch. With or without pain
2	Skin blanched. *Edema 1-6 inches.* Cool to touch. With our without pain
3	Skin blanched, *translucent. Gross edema > 6 inches.* Cool to touch. *Mild-moderate pain. Possible numbness*
4	Skin blanched, translucent. Skin tight, leaking, discolored, bruised, swollen. Gross edema > 6 inches. *Deep pitting tissue edema. Circulatory impairment. Moderate-severe pain. Infiltration of any amount of blood product, irritant, or vesicant*

Phlebitis Scale

Value	Interpretation
0	No clinical symptoms
1+	Redness with or without pain. Edema may or may not be present. No streak, no palpable cord
2+	Redness with or without pain. Edema may or may not be present. *Streak formation,* no palpable cord
3+	Redness with or without pain. Edema may or may not be present. Streak formation, *palpable cord*

Catheter Gauge Selection
- Catheter gauge selection depends on clinical factors such as prescribed therapy, diagnosis, medical history, activity level, age and status of veins
- Use the shortest length and smallest diameter catheter that will get the job done. Remember, *the smaller the catheter gauge number, the larger the diameter.*
General considerations as follows: *

Gauge	Uses	Implications
≥ 16	Large fluid/volume; rapid infusions (high-risk surgical procedures, trauma)	↑ Likelihood of pain on insertion (? anesthesia). Large vein needed. ↑ likelihood of irritation to vein wall
18	Surgery, viscous solutions (whole blood, packed RBCs). Various emergent situations	Large vein needed to accommodate catheter
20	Routine infusions and routine IV access. Minor surgical procedures	Frequently selected gauge size
22	Suitable for most infusions at slower rates. Recommended for small and/or fragile veins. Not appropriate for rapid flow rates	Easier to insert into small, thin, fragile veins but may be difficult to insert into tough skin
24, 26	Slower flow rates. Neonatal, pediatric and elderly patients	Easier to insert into extremely small veins; difficult to insert into tough skin

* Consult local institutional policies for specific guidelines and protocols as applicable

Tonicity and Fluids
- **Isotonic** Approximately same tonicity as blood plasma. Generally used for volume replacement and maintenance (D_5W, 0.9% saline)
- **Hypotonic** These solutions contain fewer particles than the solution inside the cell. Used for free water replacement (0.45% saline, Isolyte, Normosol).
- **Hypertonic** Solutions that contain a greater concentration of particles than that the cell. Used to draw excess fluid from cells and interstitial spaces (mannitol)
- **Crystalloids** Balanced salt solutions used for both maintenance and replacement therapy (0.9% saline, Lactated Ringer's, D_5W)
- **Colloids** Salt solutions containing oncotically active particles. Generally used in later stages of loss to help maintain hemodynamic stability and supplement volume (Plasmanate, Hetastarch, Dextran).

❖ Approximate adult fluid intake 50ml/kg/day. 1liter of fluid = 1kg (2.2lb.)

Nutrition

Feeding Tubes

- **Jejunal tubes** ("J" tubes). Various kinds according to how inserted. They include needle catheter jejunostomy (NCJ), percutaneous endoscopic jejunal (PEJ), and nasojejunal tubes. Usually for long-term nutritional maintenance and clients with high risk for aspiration. Verify tube placement according to institutional policy. Standard methods include aspiration of stomach contents (except for NCJ), use of external graduation marks (nasojejunal) and, X-ray

- **Gastrotomy tubes** ("G" tubes). Include percutaneous endoscopic gastric (PEG), surgical, balloon and low profile gastrostomy tubes. Verify tube placement according to institutional policy. Standard methods include use of external graduation marks, aspiration of stomach contents (in a low profile gastrostomy tube, open the anti-reflux valve first), air auscultation and X-ray

- **Nasogastric tubes** ("NG" tubes). Usually temporary, also used to aspirate stomach contents and decompress stomach. *Tube placememt:* Measure from bridge of nose to ear lobe to xiphoid process, note marking. Verify tube placement according to institutional policy. Standard methods include aspiration of stomach contents air auscultation and X-ray

❖ If in doubt about stomach contents, check pH of aspirate:
gastric pH 1.0-3.5

"Work is accomplished by those employees who have not yet reached their level of incompetence."
Laurence J. Peter "The Peter Principle"

Feeding Tube Complications and Management

Complication	Contributing factor	Management
Pulmonary aspiration	Tube in respiratory tract. Regurgitation of feeding	Verify placement prior to feeding. Add food coloring to formula to facilitate diagnosis. ↑HOB 30° during feedings. Keep ET or trache cuff inflated if possible. Ensure proper gastric emptying (aspirate prior to feeding. Generally volumes >150ml or 110-120% of hourly rate considered excessive)
Diarrhea	Meds, malnutrition, hypertonic formulas or meds, contaminated formula	Evaluate meds. Consult physician about diluting, slowing feedings, or using continuous feedings. Discard feeding containers and sets q24hr, hang formula no more than 4-8 hr unless prepackaged in sterile set. Keep open formula containers refrigerated and discard within 24hr
Constipation	Low residue formula. Low fluid intake	Consult physician about using fiber containing formulas. If no fluid restriction, ensure fluid intake is 50ml/kg/day
Gastric retention	Neural impairment or serious illness/trauma	Measure residuals q4-6hr or before feeding. Consult physician about use of "J tube." Consult physician about use of Reglan to stimulate gastric emptying. Encourage client to lie on right side unless contraindicated
Tube occlusion	Sedimentation of formula or meds	Avoid use of crushed tablets. Consult pharmacist about elixirs or suspensions. Irrigate tube with water before and after meds and feedings. Continuous feeding, irrigate q4-8hr. Use of soda or cranberry juice has been shown to coagulate whole protein tube feeding formula and may perpetuate the clog. Use of meat tenderizer is uncertain since they are not activated unless heated to high temps. Never insert a device (stylet or guidewire) into a feeding tube for unclogging. Consult physician about use of a pancreatic enzyme solution (Viokase)

Recommended Dietary Daily Allowances

Age (Yrs)	Energy (kcal)	Protein (g)	Vit A (µg RE)	Vit D (µg)	Vit E (mg α-TE)	Vit K (µg)	Vit C (mg)	Thiamin (mg)	Riboflavin (mg)	Niacin (mg NE)	Vitamin B6 (mg)	Folate (µg)	Vit B12 (µg)	Calcium (mg)	Phosphorus (mg)	Magnesium (mg)	Iron (mg)	Zinc (mg)	Iodine (µg)	Selenium (µg)
Males																				
11-14	2500	45	1000	10	10	45	50	1.3	1.5	17	1.7	150	2.0	1200	1200	270	12	15	150	40
15-18	3000	59	1000	10	10	65	60	1.5	1.8	20	2.0	200	2.0	1200	1200	400	12	15	150	50
19-24	2900	58	1000	10	10	70	60	1.5	1.7	19	2.0	200	2.0	1200	1200	350	10	15	150	70
25-50	2900	63	1000	5	10	80	60	1.5	1.7	19	2.0	200	2.0	800	800	350	10	15	150	70
51+	2300	63	1000	5	10	80	60	1.2	1.4	15	2.0	200	2.0	800	800	350	10	15	150	70
Females																				
11-14	2200	46	800	10	8	45	50	1.1	1.3	15	1.4	150	2.0	1200	1200	280	15	12	150	45
15-18	2200	44	800	10	8	55	60	1.1	1.3	15	1.5	180	2.0	1200	1200	300	15	12	150	50
19-24	2200	46	800	10	8	60	60	1.1	1.3	15	1.6	180	2.0	1200	1200	280	15	12	150	55
25-50	2200	50	800	5	8	65	60	1.1	1.3	15	1.6	180	2.0	800	800	280	15	12	150	55
51+	1900	50	800	5	8	65	60	1.0	1.2	13	1.6	180	2.0	800	800	280	10	12	150	55
Pregnant	+300	60	800	10	10	65	70	1.5	1.6	17	2.2	400	2.2	1200	1200	320	30	15	175	65
Lactating																				
1st 6 mo.	+500	65	1300	10	12	65	95	1.6	1.8	20	2.1	280	2.6	1200	1200	355	15	19	200	75
2nd 6 mo.	+500	62	1200	10	11	65	90	1.6	1.7	20	2.1	260	2.6	1200	1200	340	15	16	200	75

Determining Body Mass Index (BMI)

BMI (kg/m^2)	19	20	21	22	23	24	25	26	27	28	29	30	35	40
Height (in.)	Weight (lb.)													
58	91	96	100	105	110	115	119	124	129	134	138	143	167	191
59	94	99	104	109	114	119	124	128	133	138	143	148	173	198
60	97	102	107	112	118	123	128	133	138	143	148	153	179	204
61	100	106	111	116	122	127	132	137	143	148	153	158	185	211
62	104	109	115	120	126	131	136	142	147	153	158	164	191	218
63	107	113	118	124	130	135	141	146	152	158	163	169	197	225
64	110	116	122	128	134	140	145	151	157	163	169	174	204	232
65	114	120	126	132	138	144	150	156	162	168	174	180	210	240
66	118	124	130	136	142	148	155	161	167	173	179	186	216	247
67	121	127	134	140	146	153	159	166	172	178	185	191	223	255
68	125	131	138	144	151	158	164	171	177	184	190	197	230	262
69	128	135	142	149	155	162	169	176	182	189	196	203	236	270
70	132	139	146	153	160	167	174	181	188	195	202	207	243	278
71	136	143	150	157	165	172	179	186	193	200	208	215	250	286
72	140	147	154	162	169	177	184	191	199	206	213	221	258	294
73	144	151	159	166	174	182	189	197	204	212	219	227	265	302
74	148	155	163	171	179	186	194	202	210	218	225	233	272	311
75	152	160	168	176	184	192	200	208	216	224	232	240	279	319
76	156	164	172	180	189	197	205	213	221	230	238	246	287	328

Locate the patient's weight, in pounds, in the row to the right of his/her height, in inches. The corresponding figure at the top is the patient's BMI. A BMI of 30 or greater indicates increased risk associated with weight. For persons with added risk factors, a BMI of 27 or more indicates increased risk

Estimating Ideal Body Weight (IBW) by Gender/Height

Males		Females	
Height	Weight Allowance*	Height	Weight Allowance*
First 5 feet of height	106#	First 5 feet of height	100 #
Each added inch	Add 6#	Each added inch	Add 5#
Example: Male 5'10"	IBW = 166#	*Example*: Female 5'4"	IBW = 120#

*10% +/- allowance based on build

Relative Health Risk by BMI and Waist Size

BMI	Waist ≤ 40 inches (♂), 35 inches (♀)	Waist > 40 inches (♂), 35 inches (♀)
< 18.5		
18.5-24.9		
25.0-29.9	Increased	High
30-34.9	High	Very High
35-39.9	Very High	Very High
≥ 40	Extremely High	Extremely High

Notes:

Vitamins: Source and Action

Vitamin	Function	Source	Deficiency
A (retinol)	Production of rhodopsin (visual purple)	Liver, cream, butter, whole milk, egg yolk, green and yellow vegies, yellow fruits	Xerophthalmia
Provitamin A (carotene)	Formation and maintenance of epitheleal tissue. Toxic in large amounts		Night blindness, skin and mucous membrane infections, faulty tooth formation
D	Absorption of Calcium and phosphorus. Toxic in large amounts	Fish oils, fortified milk	Rickets, faulty bone growth, osteomalacia in adults
E	Antioxidant with Vit. A and unsaturated fatty acids. Hemopoiesis, reproduction	Vegetable oils	Hemolysis of RBCs, possible protection of unsaturated fatty acids
K	Blood clotting. Toxic in large amounts	Green leafy vegetables, cheese, egg yolk, liver	Bleeding tendencies, poor coagulation
C	Collagen and fibrous tissue formation, aids in fighting bacterial infections	Citrus fruits, tomatoes, green leafy vegetables	Scurvy, bruising, megaloblastic anemia
Thiamin B_1	Carbohydrate metabolism	Pork, beef, liver, whole grains, legumes	Beriberi
Riboflavin B_2	Nutrient metabolism, prevents cataracts	Milk, liver, cheese, eggs, green leafy veggies	Cheilosis, local inflammation, desquamation, glossitis

Vitamins: Source and Action (cont.)

Vitamin	Function	Source	Deficiency
Niacin	Involved in ATP metabolism	Meat, peanuts, enriched grains	Pellagra
Pyridoxine B_6	Amino acid metabolism	Wheat, corn, meat, liver	Hypochromic microcytic anemia
Folic Acid B_9	Essential for cell growth and reproduction	Spinach and other green leafy veggies, liver, lima beans, nuts	Poor growth, graying hair, glossitis, stomatitis, need for folic acid increased in pregnacy, infancy and by stress
Cobalamin B_{12}	Coenzyme in protein synthesis	Liver, meat, egg, cheese	Extrinsic factor in pernicious anemia

Cholesterol Recommendations (Lipids)

LDL Cholesterol	Triglycerides
<100 Optimal	<150 mg/dL Normal
100-129 Near optimal/above optimal	150-199 mg/dL Borderline-high
130-159 Borderline high	200-499 mg/dL High
160-189 High	≥500 mg/dL Very high
≥190 Very high	

Total Cholesterol	HDL Cholesterol
<200 Desirable	<40 Low
200-239 Borderline high	≥60 High
≥240 High	

"We boil at different degrees."
Ralph Waldo Emerson

Notes:

Basic Life Support*

Cardiopulmonary Resuscitation (CPR)

- Determine if unresponsive
- Activate EMS (call 911), get automated external defibrillator (AED)[1]
- Open airway, check for breathing (look, listen and feel)[2]
- If not breathing give 2 slow breaths[3] and check circulation (pulse)[4]
- If no pulse begin compressions (see chart below) until AED arrives
- Reassess after 4 compression/ventilation cycles by checking pulse
- If no pulse/no signs of circulation, continue CPR
- If signs of circulation are present, check breathing. If inadequate breathing, continue rescue breathing 1 breath every 5 seconds
- If breathing is adequate, place in a recovery position and monitor

See *CPR Notes* in the following page

Compressions

	Adult	Child	Infant
Pulse Check	Carotid artery	Carotid artery	Brachial artery
Hand Position	Two hands, lower half of sternum (use heel of hand)	One hand, lower half of sternum (use heel of hand)	Two fingers, lower half of sternum (one finger width below nipple line). "Two thumb encircling" hand technique is preferred for 2 rescuer CPR
Compression Depth	1.5"-2"	1"-1.5"	0.5"-1"
Cycle (compression : breath)	15:2 (1 or 2 rescuer CPR)	5:1 (1 or 2 rescuer CPR)	5:1 (1 or 2 rescuer CPR). Newborns or premature infants in the neonatal ICU 3:1
Rate	Approximately 100 comp/min.	Approximately 100 comp/min.	*At least* 100 comp/min

* Source: Guidelines 2000 for CPR and ECC, American Heart Association

Basic Life Support Notes

- **[1]Getting Help**
  Generally, 3 actions must occur at once at the scene of a cardiac arrest: Activation of EMS (or resuscitation team in a hospital), CPR and use of AED. When 2 or more rescuers are present, these actions can be initiated simultaneously (see *Automated External Defibrillator* Section on the following pages for AED use).

  " Phone first" to activate EMS as soon as emergency is recognized. If victim is <8 years old, then "phone fast" (begin CPR for approximately 1 minute then activate EMS). Exceptions include:
  1. Near-drowning, "phone fast," all ages
  2. Arrest associated with trauma, "phone fast," all ages
  3. Drug overdoses, "phone fast," all ages
  4. Cardiac arrest in children known to be at high risk for arrhythmias, "phone first," all ages

- **[2]Airway**
  Use the "head tilt-chin lift" technique. Use the "jaw-thrust" technique if there is a suspected spine injury.

- **[3]Breathing**
  Deliver mouth-to mouth or mouth-to-mask rescue breaths over 2 seconds to reduce risk of gastric inflation. If unable to ventilate, reposition, reopen airway and attempt to ventilate again. If still unable to ventilate, consider foreign body airway obstruction: Perform Heimlich maneuver (abdominal thrusts) up to 5 times, open the airway using the "tongue-jaw lift," perform a finger sweep to remove foreign object and attempt to ventilate. Repeat until obstruction is cleared or other procedures are available to establish a patent airway. The finger sweep is to be used only on the unresponsive-unconscious adult with a complete foreign body airway obstruction. For child and infant victims: look in mouth, if no foreign bodies are visible do not perform finger sweep, if foreign bodies are visible you may remove them.

- **[4]Circulation**
  Signs of circulation include normal breathing, coughing or movement. Pulse check should take no more than 10 seconds.

Automated External Defibrillator (AED)

The *American Heart Association* recommends that healthcare providers with a duty to perform CPR be trained, equipped, and authorized to perform defibrillation. In healthcare facilities, healthcare providers should be able to deliver a shock within 3+/-1 minutes of arrest. AED use is considered a basic life support skill

AED: Special Situations

- **Water** Remove patient from freestanding water and dry the patient's chest before use
- **Children** Not recommended for use in infants and children <8 years old
- **Transdermal Medications** Do not place electrodes directly over medication patch. Remove medication patch and wipe area clean before electrode placement
- **Implanted Pacemakers and Defibrillators (ICDs)** Place electrode pad at least 1 inch away from implanted device. If ICD is delivering shocks to victim, allow 30-60 seconds for it to complete its treatment cycle. The analysis and shock cycles of ICDs and AEDs may conflict

AED: Operation of "Universal AED"

1. Power On

2. Attach Electrode Pads Upper-right sternal border (below clavicle) and lateral to the left nipple (a few inches below axilla)

3. Press "Analyze" Button If the device is equipped with one, some devices will analyze automatically. The device will analyze the cardiac rhythm (5-15 seconds). If ventricular fibrillation or a rapid ventricular tachycardia is present, an alarm or message (visual or auditory) will announce that "shock is indicated." If not, "no shock indicated" will be displayed

4. Clear Patient and Shock Ensure everyone is clear (no one is in contact with patient). Press "shock" button. Do not start CPR after first shock. AEDs are programmed to deliver up to 3 shocks, if needed, followed by a pause. Some models do this automatically, others may require that you press "Analyze" after the shock

AED and CPR

- Continue CPR until AED arrives (see page 29)
- Power "On," attach electrode pads and attempt to defibrillate (Analyze, "Clear," Shock, "Clear") up to 3 times if advised (see page 31)
- After 3 shocks or after any "no shock indicated" message, check for signs of circulation (pulse)
- If no signs of circulation, perform CPR for 1 minute
- Check for signs of circulation and if absent continue with use of AED as prompted: Analyze, "Clear," Shock, "Clear." Repeat up to 3 shocks, then another minute of CPR if needed etc.
- If signs of circulation are present, check breathing. If inadequate breathing: continue rescue breathing 1 breath every 5 seconds
- If breathing is adequate, place in a recovery position and monitor

"It may seem a strange principle to enunciate as the very first requirement in a hospital that it should do the sick no harm"
Florence Nightingale

Notes:

Medications

Dosage Formulas

- **Amount to Administer**

(Dose ordered / Dose on hand) x Amount on hand = Amount to administer
   e.g. Order: 100mg Theophylline po q6h. Have 200mg per tablet.
   (100/200) = 0.5 X 1 tablet = 0.5 (1/2 tablet)

- **Hourly Rate**

   Total volume / Total # of hours infusing = Hourly rate
   e.g. Order: Infuse 1000ml NaCl over 12 hours
   1000/12 = 83.3 ml/hr (pump rate)

- **Determine Drops per Minute**

   (Total volume x Drop factor) / Time in minutes = Drops per minute
   Drop Factor: Microdrip Infusion Set: 60gtt/min.
                Macrodrip Infusion Set: 15gtt/min.
If in doubt, look at the infusion set package, it will tell you the drop factor
   e.g. Order: Infuse 1000ml NaCl over 12 hours
   (83.3X60)/60 = 83gtt/min or same order with a macrodrip
   (83.3X 15)/60 = 21gtt/min

- **Determine Concentration**

   e.g. Order: IV fluids have 25,000 units of Heparin in 500cc of ½ NS.
   25,000u/500cc = 50 units/cc

- **To Determine Rate for Dose per Hour**

   e.g. Order: Administer 90 mg of Theophylline per hour. The IV fluids hanging are 1000mg of Theophylline in 250cc of D5 ½ NS.
   Concentration = 1000mg/250cc = 4mg/cc
   Dose per hour = 90 mg per hour/4mg per cc = 22.5 cc (rate for pump)

Notes:

Syringe Compatibility

Locate first drug on left column. Note the appropriate number of second drug and find its location along the top row. Compatibility is found on the grid square where the name of the first drug and the number of the second drug meet

	1	2	3	4	5	6	7	8	9	10	11	12	13	14	15	16	17	18	19
Atropine (1)		C		I	C	C		C	C	C	C	C	C	C	C	C	C	I	
Butorphanol (2) *Stadol*	C			I	C		I	C	C	C	C	C	I	C	C		C	I	C
Codeine (3)				I													I		I
Diazepam (4) *Valium*	I	I	I		I	I		I	I	I		I	I	I	I		I	I	I
Fentanyl (5)	C	C		I		C		C	C	C		C	I	C	C	C	C	I	
Glycopyrrolate (6) *Robinul*	C			I	C			C	C				C	I	C	C	C	I	
Heparin (7)		I		I					I			I		I			I		
Hydroxyzine (8) *Atarax, Vistaril*	C	C		I	C	C			C	C		C	I	C	C	I	C	I	
Meperidine (9) *Demerol, Pethadol*	C	C		I	C	C	I	C		C		I	I	C	C	C	C	I	
Metoclopramide (10) *Reglan, Maxolon*	C	C		I	C			C	C			C		C	C	C	C	I	
Midazolam (11) *Versed*	C	C			C	C		C	C			C	I	I	C	I	C	I	C
Morphine (12)	C	C		I	C	C	I	C	I	C			I	C	C	C	C	I	
Pentobarbital (13) *Nembutal*	C	I	I	I	I	I		I	I		I	I		I	I	I	C	I	
Prochlorperazine (14) *Compazine*	C	C		I	C	C		C	C	C		C	I		C	C	C	I	
Promethazine (15) *Phenergan*	C	C		I	C	C		C	C	C	C	C	I	C			C	I	
Ranitidine (16) *Zantac*	C				C	C		I	C	C	I	C		C	C			C	C
Scopolamine Hbr (17)	C	C		I	C	C		C	C	C	C	C	C	C	C	C		I	
Secobarbital (18)	I	I	I	I	I	I		I	I	I		I	I	I	I		I		I
Thiethylperazine (19) *Torecan*		C		I											C		I		

C = Compatible
I = Incompatible
☐ = No documented information

Common trade names in *Italics*

"The greatest evil is physical pain."
St Augustine

Commonly Used Analgesics in Adults*

Acetaminophen (Tylenol) PO 325-650mg q4 (max 1g/qid)	**Fentanyl citrate** Preop:IM/IV 0.05-0.1mg q30-60min. Postop:IM 0.05-0.1mg q1-2hr prn
Acetaminophen & codeine PO15-60mg codeine q4 (max 360mg codeine/day)	**Ibuprofen** (Advil, Motrin, Nuprin) 200-400mg q4-6 hr (max 1,200mg/day)
Amitriptyline hydrochloride (Elavil) chronic pain PO 50-100 mg/day	**Meperidine HCL** (Demerol) PO/IM/SC 50-100 mgq3-4hr, continuous IV: 15-35mg/hr
Acetaminophen & hydrocodone (Lorcet 10/650) PO 1 tabs q4-6hr (max 6 tabs/24hr)	**Morphine** IM/SC 10-20mg/70kg q4h. IV 2.5-15mg/70kg in 4-5ml H_2O over 4-5min
Aspirin PO 325-600mg q4	**Naproxen** (Naprosyn) mild to moderate pain, initial 550mg then 275mg q6-8hr prn (max 1,375mg/day)
Codeine sulfate PO/IV/IM, SC 15-60mg q4-6hr (max 360mg/qd)	**Oxycodone HCL** (OxyContin, Roxicodone) PO 10-30mg q4hr individualized dose

Insulin Preparations*

Type of Insulin	Time of onset (hr)	Peak of action (hr)	Duration of action (hr)	Appearance
Rapid acting				
Lispro (Humalog)	15 min	40-60 min	46 min half-life	Clear
Regular	<1	2-4	4-6	Clear
Crystalline zinc	<1	2-4	5-8	Clear
Semilente	1-2	3-10	10-16	Cloudy
Intermediate				
NPH	1-2	4-12	18-24	Cloudy
Globin zinc	2-4	6-10	12-18	Clear
Lente	1-3	6-15	18-24	Cloudy
Slow acting				
Protamine zinc	4-8	14-24	36+	Cloudy
Ultralente	4-8	10-30	28-36	Cloudy

*Consult a drug reference guide for further specific information including contraindications, interactions and other nursing clinical concerns.

Notes:

NANDA Nursing Diagnoses*

*By permission, *Nursing Diagnoses: Definitions & Classification 2001-2002 NANDA*

- **Exchanging**

Imbalanced nutrition: More than body requirements
Imbalanced nutrition: Less than body requirements
Risk for imbalanced nutrition: More than body requirements
Risk for infection
Risk for imbalanced body temperature
Hypothermia
Hyperthermia
Ineffective thermoregulation
Autonomic dysreflexia
Risk for autonomic dysreflexia
Constipation
Perceived constipation
Diarrhea
Bowel incontinence
Risk for constipation
Impaired urinary elimination
Stress urinary incontinence
Reflex urinary incontinence
Urge urinary incontinence
Functional urinary incontinence
Total urinary incontinence
Risk for urge urinary incontinence
Urinary retention
Ineffective tissue perfusion (specify type: renal, cerebral, cardiopulmonary, gastrointestinal, peripheral)

(Exchanging cont.)

Risk for fluid volume imbalance
Excess fluid volume
Deficient fluid volume
Risk for deficient fluid volume
Decreased cardiac output
Impaired gas exchange
Ineffective airway clearance
Ineffective breathing pattern
Impaired spontaneous ventilation
Dysfunctional ventilatory weaning response
Risk for injury
Risk for suffocation
Risk for poisoning
Risk for trauma
Risk for aspiration
Risk for disuse syndrome
Latex allergy response
Risk for latex allergy response
Ineffective protection
Impaired tissue integrity
Impaired oral mucous membrane
Impaired skin integrity
Risk for impaired skin integrity
Impaired dentition
Decreased intracranial adaptive capacity
Disturbed energy field

- **Communicating**

Impaired verbal communication

- 37 -

NANDA Nursing Diagnoses (cont.)

- **Relating**
Impaired social interaction
Social isolation
Risk for loneliness
Ineffective role performance
Deficient parenting
Risk for deficient parenting
Risk for impaired parent/infant/child attachment
Sexual dysfunction
Interrupted family processes
Caregiver role strain
Risk for caregiver role strain
Altered family processes: Alcoholism
Parental role conflict
Ineffective sexuality patterns

- **Valuing**
Spiritual distress
Risk for spiritual distress
Readiness for enhanced spiritual well-being

- **Choosing**
Ineffective coping
Impaired adjustment
Defensive coping
Ineffective denial
Disabled family coping
Compromised family coping
Readiness for enhanced family coping
Readiness for enhanced community coping

(Choosing cont.)
Ineffective community coping
Ineffective therapeutic regimen management
Noncompliance (specify)
Ineffective family therapeutic regimen management
Ineffective community therapeutic regimen management
Effective therapeutic regimen management
Decisional conflict (specify)
Health-seeking behaviors (specify)

- **Moving**
Impaired physical mobility
Risk for peripheral neurovascular dysfunction
Risk for perioperative-positioning injury
Impaired walking
Impaired wheelchair mobility
Impaired transfer ability
Impaired bed mobility
Activity intolerance
Fatigue
Risk for activity intolerance
Sleep pattern disturbance
Sleep deprivation
Deficient diversional activity
Impaired home maintenance
Ineffective health maintenance
Delayed surgical recovery
Adult failure to thrive

NANDA Nursing Diagnoses (cont.)

(Moving cont.)
Feeding self-care deficit
Impaired swallowing
Ineffective breastfeeding
Interrupted breastfeeding
Effective breastfeeding
Ineffective infant feeding pattern
Bathing/hygiene self-care deficit
Dressing/grooming self-care deficit
Toileting self-care deficit
Delayed growth and development
Risk for delayed development
Risk for disproportionate growth
Relocation stress syndrome
Risk for disorganized infant behavior
Disorganized infant behavior
Readiness for enhanced organized infant behavior

- **Perceiving**

Disturbed body image
Disturbed self-esteem
Chronic low self-esteem
Situational low self-esteem
Disturbed personal identity
Disturbed sensory perception (specify: visual, auditory, kinesthetic, gustatory, tactile, olfactory)
Unilateral neglect
Hopelessness
Powerlessness

- **Knowing**

Deficient knowledge (specify)
Impaired environmental interpretation syndrome

(Knowing cont.)
Acute confusion
Chronic confusion
Disturbed thought processes
Impaired memory

- **Feeling**

Acute pain
Chronic pain
Nausea
Dysfunctional grieving
Anticipatory grieving
Chronic sorrow
Risk for other-directed violence
Risk for self-mutilation
Risk for self-directed violence
Post-trauma syndrome
Rape-trauma syndrome
Rape-trauma syndrome: Compound reaction
Rape-trauma syndrome: Silent reaction
Risk for post-trauma syndrome
Anxiety
Death anxiety
Fear

- **New Nursing Dx, April 2000**

Risk for relocation stress syndrome
Risk for suicide
Self-mutilation
Risk for powerlessness
Risk for situational low self-esteem
Wandering
Risk for falls

References

American Heart Association (2000). *Guidelines 2000 for CPR and ECC.* Dallas, TX: American Heart Association.

Anderson N. K. (Ed.). (2002). *Mosby's Medical, Nursing & Allied Health Dictionary.* (6th ed.). Philadelphia, PA: WB Saunders.

Hankins J. et al (2001). *Infusion Therapy in Clinical Practice.* Philadelphia, PA: Harcourt Health Sciences.

Hospital Infections Program (1999). *Exposure to Blood; What Healthcare Workers Need to Know.* Atlanta, GA: Centers for Disease Control and Prevention.

Jarvis, C. (2000). *Physical Examination and Health Assessment* (3rd ed.). Philadelphia, PA: WB Saunders.

LeFever, J. K. (1999). *Laboratory and Diagnostic Tests with Nursing Implications.* (5th ed.). Stamford, CT: Appleton & Lange.

National Heart, Lung, and Blood Institute. (2001). *Third Report of the National Cholesterol Education Program.* (Publication No. 01-3670). Bethesda, MD: National Institutes of Health.

North American Nursing Diagnosis Association. (2001). *NANDA Nursing Diagnosis: Definitions and Classifications 2000-2002.* (Philadelphia, PA: NANDA

Spratto, G. & Woods, A. (2002). *2003 PDR Nurse's Drug Handbook.* Clifton Park, NY: Delmar Learning

Swartz, H. M. (2001). *Textbook of Physical Diagnosis: History and Examination.* (4th ed.). Philadelphia, PA: WB Saunders.

Urden, D. L. et al (2001). *Thelan's Critical Care nursing: Diagnosis and Management,* (4th ed.). St. Louis, MO: Mosby.

U.S. Public Health Service (2001). *Updated Guidelines for the Management of Occupational Exposures to HBV, HCV, and HIV and Recommendations for Postexposure Prophylaxis.* Washington DC: U.S. Public Health Service.